Grandma's Natural Remedies and Ancient Herbal Beauty Recipes

Volume 2

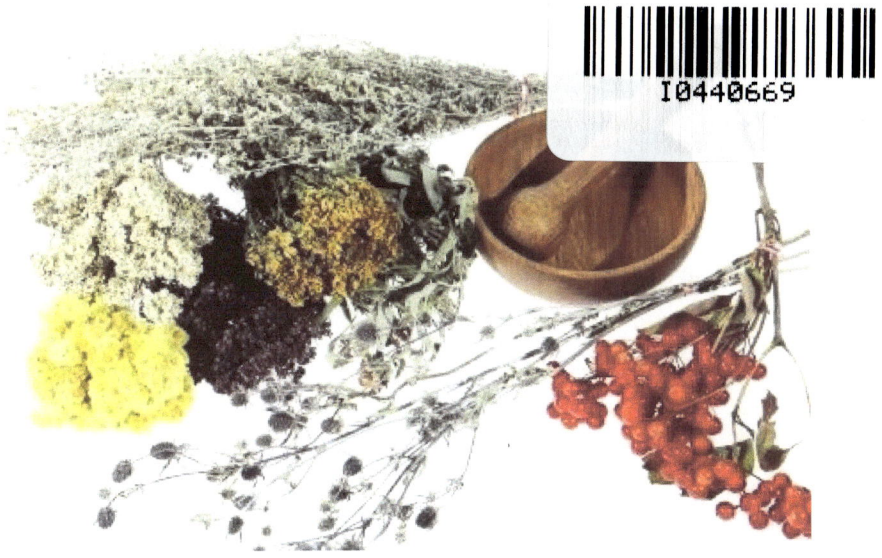

Dueep J Singh

Natural Remedy Series

Mendon Cottage Books

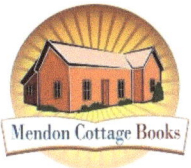

JD-Biz Publishing

Download Free Books!

http://MendonCottageBooks.com

Disclaimer

The information is this book is provided for informational purposes only. It is not intended to be used and medical advice or a substitute for proper medical treatment by a qualified health care provider. The information is believed to be accurate as presented based on research by the author.

The contents have not been evaluated by the U.S. Food and Drug Administration or any other Government or Health Organization and the contents in this book are not to be used to treat cure or prevent disease.

The author or publisher is not responsible for the use or safety of any diet, procedure or treatment mentioned in this book. The author or publisher is not responsible for errors or omissions that may exist.

Warning

The Book is for informational purposes only and before taking on any diet, treatment or medical procedure it is recommended to consult with your primary health care provider.

Our books are available at

1. Amazon.com

2. Barnes and Noble

3. Itunes

4. Kobo

5. Smashwords

6. Google Play Books

Table of Contents

Introduction 5

Rules for Staying Healthy [With My Views, Opinions, and Experience] 9

Remedies for Different Ailments 15

Piles 15

Hemorrhoids 15

Constipation 16

Flatulence 16

What Is Black Salt? 16

Where can you get black salt? 17

Migraine 18

Oh, Those Pearlies... (Tooth and mouth care).....................................20

Ulcers in your mouth...22

Drooling/Excess salivation 23

Toothache powder...23

Sensitive teeth..23

The Magic of Face Masks 25

Aloe Vera Gel...27

How to Make Your Own Personalized Face Masks..............................27

Masks for a dry skin 28

Tomato mask..29

Oily skin can be treated with these masks...............................30

    What is Fuller's earth? 30

Orange mask 30

Normal skins can be treated by these masks............................31

Honey mask...31

cucumber and milk mask 31

Appendix: 34

How to make salty lassi to prevent dehydration in summer 34

Mattha – spicy lassi 34

How to make jalebis dripping in sugar syrup 34

How to make Desi Ghee (clarified butter) 36

How to make Rose water (Gulab Jal) 37

Conclusion..39

Author Bio 40

Publisher 51

Introduction

Somebody asked me once why I did not become a doctor and then join the Defense Services as a Doctor like the majority of my family members? Here was I with an easily obtained Degree in Natural Sciences and all my knowledge -garnered during a peripatetic childhood and youth-about natural remedies, ancient medicine and natural healing processes.

The medical or the engineering fields were the only options left for good students, during the time I was at University. And I give them my stock answer, which I consider logical and sensible, "If I become a doctor, I will be giving my patients chemical-based medicine, and I will just be curing their bodies. On the other hand, if I stick to my habit of learning more about natural remedies and ancient remedies, I will be curing their bodies, as well as fighting the disease from the root onwards."

My grandmother had learned about natural remedies and beauty recipes from her grandmother, and this wisdom was passed down the ages, from mother to daughter. For millenniums, every mother in every ancient civilization taught her daughters the rudimentary art of survival and staying beautiful and youthful with fruits, vegetables, spices, and herbs. This is now considered to be alternative medicine by doctors in the West. But this was the medicine with which people survived through centuries and stayed healthy.

So if you believe in natural remedies, and naturopathic treatments, the cures are right around you. But many of us would rather go to a doctor and get some expensive medicine. The side effect of that medicine is going to be that some other part of our system is going to get affected. After that we go back to the doctor again and get some medicine to treat that side effect. That medicine produces another side effect. This is going to be your way of living for the rest of your life. However, if you eat natural medicines, you are never going to suffer from any sort of side effects. That is because natural products are more tuned to your body's systems and natural needs, than chemical drugs are.

Chemical drugs are short term healers. Natural medicines go in for healing your body permanently.

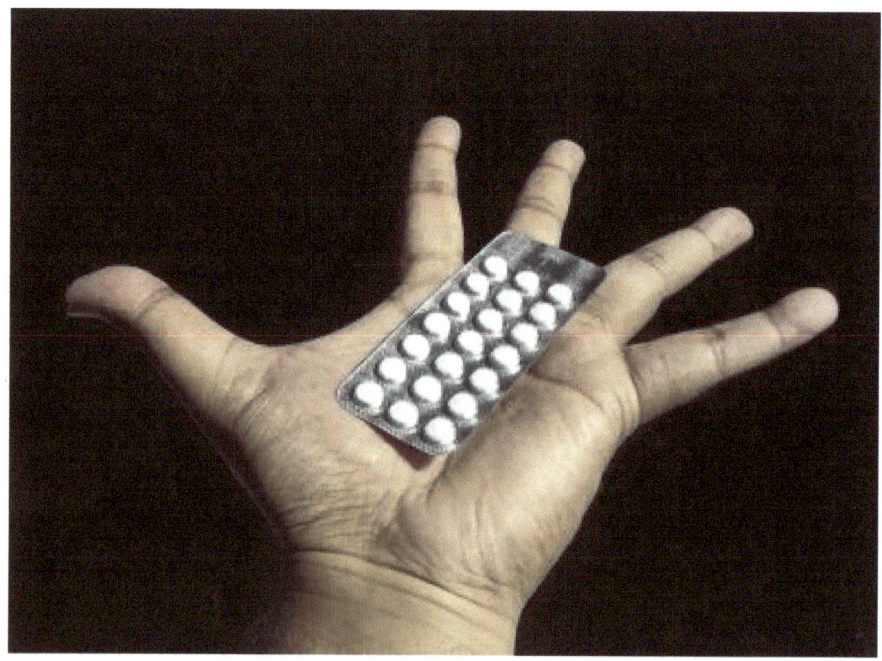

Say no to chemical drugs, as much as possible

For all those who have read Lloyd C Douglas' <u>Magnificent Obsession</u> and liked it, Mr. Douglas had some more words spoken by another of his popular characters, in "Disputed Passage". That doctor said something on the lines of – it is not our duty to just cure the body. We have to cure the mind and spirit too and heal them", much to the disgust of doctor Tubby Forrester, who considered every human to be a machine which needed to be put right, and where did emotions and spirit and soul come into this curing process?

At the end of the story, Dr. Forrester had to accept the fact that human beings had to be treated by doctors who understood their psychological, mental, spiritual and emotional makeup. Unfortunately, this is not being done today, because doctors are harried, and have to see a number of patients till the end of a day. Their hearts are set in giving the patients quick relief medicines which are going to give them temporary relief, and then they will need to come back again for the next dose of treatments.

That was not what I wanted out of life.

This was definitely not what the ancient wise men preached. Their idea was to tackle the disease from the roots, and get rid of it permanently. Look at any ancient civilization's medical history – Chinese, Japanese, Mesopotamian, Greek, Indian, Mayan – you name it, each ancient doctor knew that the remedy could only work when the heart, mind, spirit, soul and body was in perfect harmony, and in tune.

So, this book is for all of us who want to preserve the teachings of the ancient wise men, brought down to us by word of mouth. These are time tested and effective remedies, which work. So if you are looking for best and effective natural remedies with natural products, you are going to enjoy the knowledge brought to you in this book.

This book is based on a collection of ancient remedies and beauty recipes, collected from grandma's reminiscences, – and not only mine, a multitude of grandmas, grandpas, experienced Hakims, shamans, Vaids, and other wise men, and also well-known ancient beauties well-versed in ancient healing lore brought down through the ages from India, Greece, Persia, Turkey, and Uzbekistan to benefit mankind globally.

Not all of these remedies are going to be of herbal medicines. Some of them are going to be about natural healing creams with chemical antiseptics like sulfa drugs and boric acid for external use and some are going to be with food recipes, which cure.

Rules for Staying Healthy [With My Views, Opinions, and Experience]

The ancients had very strict rules about staying healthy, and these rules had to be practiced by them. According to them these rules had been set out by their teachers, and passed down from master to pupil and if some of them sound obsolete or even laughable in the hectic lifestyle of the 21st century, here they are.

Wake up at Dawn. Wash your mouth out and then drink one glass of fresh water. [Waking up at Dawn is strictly for the birds for me, but the ancients did that, because they thought that not a moment of the precious day should be wasted.]

In olden days, you had utensils made out of copper. People stored water in them, and I think that this was a good way in which you could get necessary minerals in your body. So if you have a copper pot anywhere or a copper jug, fill it up with drinking water at night, and drink that water down first thing in the morning. This prevents constipation and gets your alimentary canal moving. [I tried this out for three days, and I definitely did not suffer from any sort of constipation, running to the bathroom within the next half hour but then I forgot about this way to keep healthy in the daily rush to get ready in order to reach the office in time.]

This was a rule which I found rather funny, but it is still being practiced by people in rural India. Clench your teeth when you are emptying out your bowels. Supposedly, this fixes your teeth, and you are never going to suffer from shaking teeth ever again. I am being a little bit risqué here, but I bet they clenched their teeth automatically if they were suffering from constipation and were trying to get their system and clear of all that accumulated stuff. Even so, what is so difficult about clenching your teeth, and if it really sets the more firmly in your gums, so much the better.

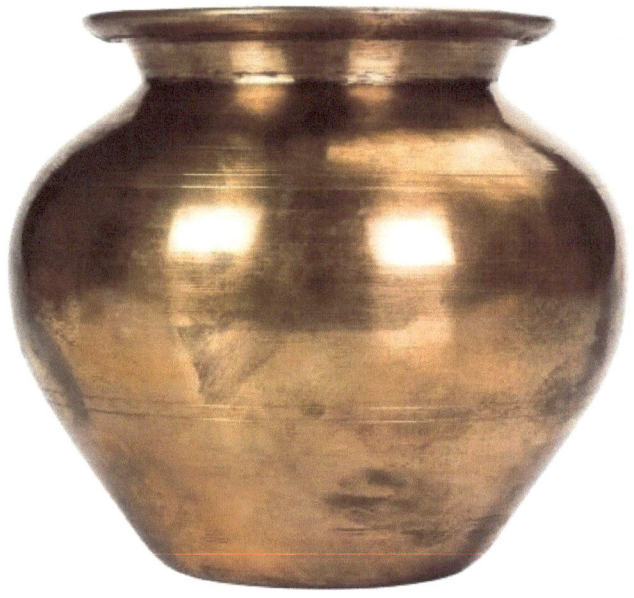

These copper pots are normally called Kalashes and are often used in religious rituals, in India.

While washing your hands and face, fill your mouth up with water while you are splashing water in your eyes. This strengthens the power of your eyes.

Drink one glass of water before you begin the meal. Do not drink water while eating your meal. But if the spices make your eyes water, then just take one sip of water, or one spoonful of yogurt to cool down your system. Drink as much water as you like, one hour after you have had your meal. That means that your tummy has had time to mix the meal, with its digestive enzymes and acids and the water drunk after an hour is going to make that mixture more easily assimilated in to your system.

Remember to do a little bit of walking after a meal. Drink a glass of warm milk with honey before you go to sleep after washing your face, hands and feet. [Now this washing idea is sensible – no dirty feet means no dirty sheets! But in reality, the scrubbing you do on your feet is a sort of feet massage, which is going to reduce tension and stress in your body and make you relax.]

I do not know whether this has been scientifically proven or not, but a person suffering from diabetes, running, morning and evening is going to find the elimination of sugar in urine significantly reduced.

All right, this has nothing to do with natural remedies, but this is a rule for keeping healthy, especially for those people who drink alcohol, and suffer from hangovers. I am hundred percent sure that in ancient times, all of them knew everything about hangovers, and how to prevent them, and how to get rid of them too.

So if you are going to a party, drink the white of an egg to coat your tummy lining, and mix your round of drinks with glasses of water or fresh juice, so that your body still keeps hydrated and then eat a whole lemon when you go home. Drink a glass of warm lemon juice before you drop off to sleep. No hangovers ever.

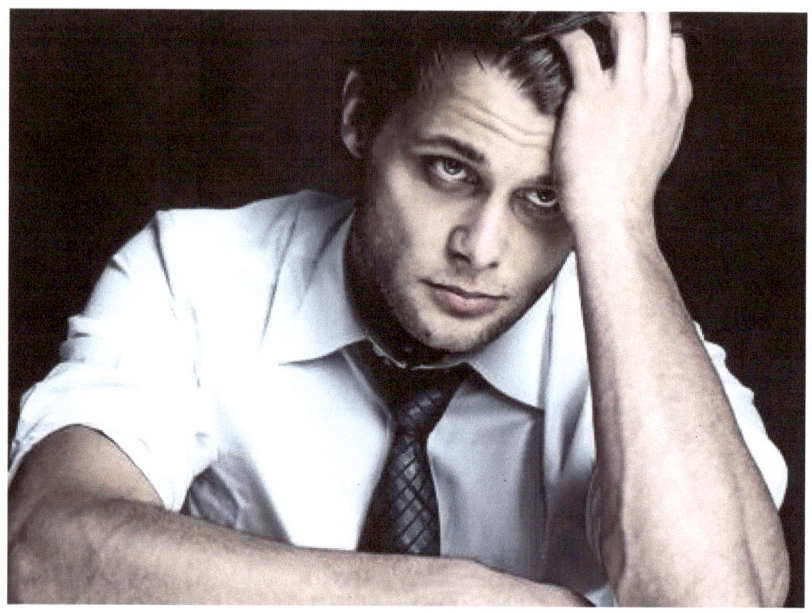

After effect of heavy drinking last night?

This reminds me of the one and only time when I drank hard alcohol, – I am a natural teetotaler, not even drinking tea and coffee – because my really decent office pals had decided that the New Year had to be ushered in at the party with lots of drinks, plenty of food and lots of good cheer and beer.

Naturally, I kept saying "no, I do not drink, and I have never drunk any hard alcohol," till one mischievous colleague said "okay, have fruit punch, DJ". Never having drunk alcohol beforehand, I did not know that the fruit juices had been doctored with nearly odorless gin, a bit of moonshine and vodka in large quantities. And I think I was too naïve to understand that they wanted DJ to get thoroughly soused and start singing arias from Carmen or dance on the tabletop or dive into the swimming pool fully clothed. Which I do not do in my normal senses.

(Luckily, thanks to this white of an egg recipe, given to me by my grandfather, – who had to take part in lots of social drinking as an Army officer in the 30s, 40s and 50s – "All knowledge is useful, my child, even if you never use it ever in your life, white of an egg and lots of water/soda/fresh fruit juice, if you find any, in between drinks." I had the best New Year's party I ever had.")

Well, you can imagine what happened. Here I was, gulping drinks down, and saying, "really delicious, that is nice, can I have some more please," without any hint of slurring, while all the rest were finding it difficult to walk in a straight line. Also, there were no chances of me breaking out into *"Votre toast je peux vous le rendre, senors, senors…Toreador en garde…"* Or perhaps an energetic Bhangra or Kuchipudi on the table among the leftovers.*)*

The next morning, everybody had a terrible hangover and was thinking about the best way to murder me, especially when I opened up the windows of the office, spoke to them in a bright, cheery, loud tone, and also told them what I was going to have for lunch, fried bacon with huge Hoagies for starters with chips smothered in tomato sauce and mustard, topped off with rich chocolate pastry or perhaps a nice rich creamy meringue or a jelly and custard soufflé? Mmmmm? And should I bring some back for any of them? One muttered that he would really kill me when he felt a bit better. After slow roasting on a barbecue, while being basted with gin, vodka and fruit punch.

Some of them still have not forgiven me for the misery I put them through, even though we laugh over it whenever we talk – alas, only on New Year, how time does fly –. Also, thanks to this natural ancient remedy they are now under the impression that a majority of their Indian or even other Eastern colleagues, -even those who pretend they do not drink and methinks they protesteth too much, the sly hypocrites holding out on secret remedies for their best buddies - are hard topers, who can just pour down drinks and still come up fresh as a daisy in the morning, bright eyed and bushy tailed. To make others contemplate justified homicide or pesticide.

I would not advise you to go in for a hard drinking session every day, just because I have given you these remedies. Nevertheless, now that the holiday season is coming in, and you will be drinking with your friends and colleagues to the New Year, I have given you this natural remedy solution, given to me by my grandfather. So consider this to be grandfathers' remedies too.

The last rule for healthy living – do not go to sleep him immediately after drinking hot milk, tea or coffee. Let your body relax a little.

Remedies for Different Ailments

Piles

Piles is a condition which normally affects people suffering from constipation. Piles is normally caused by hemorrhoids in the anal region. Sometimes the hemorrhoids burst when a patient is undergoing bowel movements. This causes the passage of blood to be eliminated along with the feces. This is naturally going to cause patients a lot of concern.

If a patient is suffering from piles, his digestive system is going to go awry. He may not feel hungry, and he may get constipated. He may suffer from flatulence. This affects the digestive system as well as the kidneys, liver and heart adversely. The patient may also have mild facial swelling.

Do not eat meat, grapes, and mangoes. When you are suffering from piles, alcohol is forbidden. Eating green leafy vegetables to prevent constipation is advised.

Hemorrhoids

Here is a **cream** with which you can get relief from hemorrhoids. This has some ingredients which do not come in natural remedies, like boric acid and sulfadiazine. Nevertheless, this is an effective way in which you can get rid of hemorrhoids.

50 g white Vaseline petroleum jelly, 6 g camphor tablets, three tablets sulfadiazine, 6 g boric acid powder. Powder them all together. Apply on hemorrhoids; – both inside and outside, this is a messy process – before going to sleep at night and before going to the toilet in the morning.

If the hemorrhoids have burst and blood appears with the feces, try this remedy –

Take 10 g of Marigold green leaves – I guess they will not be more than two – three leaves, four at the most – 1 ½ teaspoons when ground –,five peppercorns, 10 g of sugar candy/rock sugar – known as kuja Mishri-and grind them in 60 g water. Drink this mixture once a day for four days. This is going to get rid of blood in piles.

Constipation

Constipation is an extremely common ailment. So the next time you find your stomach bloating, you suffering from flatulence, and you troubled with indigestion, all you have to do is mix up one and a half teaspoons each of bishops weed, fennel seeds, and black salt with 1 teaspoon of pepper. Powder them together and put them in one glass of water. Drink down. This is going to cure your constipation.

Flatulence

Try drinking Mattha [recipe given in appendix] after every meal. Not only is this going to keep you healthy, but it is going to pep up your digestive system. This Mattha is going to have two pinches of bishops weed and a pinch of black salt. Drink it with/after every meal.

What Is Black Salt?

Some of my Western friends said that black salt, reminded them of rotten eggs. This salt has a lot of sulfide in it. It is because of this sulfide, that it is used to spice up street food. In India, and other parts of with the Indian subcontinent, this is a part of every kitchen, especially when you want to spice up meat, or any dish to make it more spicy and tangy. Its side effects on your health are negligible, so I normally use rock salt and black salt instead of sea salt in my food. So if you are looking for a salt free diet, because your doctor recommended it due to high sodium content, but you still cannot do without salt, try, rock salt, or black salt. Why stop enjoying delicious food, just because you cannot eat salt?

http://en.wikipedia.org/wiki/Kala_Namak

Where can you get black salt?
Black salt is easily available in powdered form or in solid form online, or in Asian grocery shops. Ask for Kala Namak.(*Kaalaa Nuh-muh-k)* Rocksalt is pinkish in color and is mined in salt beds. You can call this Sendha (*Say-n-dhaa- Nuhmuhk*). Ordinary sea salt is just namak -nuhmuhk.

Buy this from Amazon. Bargains start from USD3.48. Remember that this is a salt. So when you use this, do not use sea salt. It is either – or.

http://www.amazon.com/Black-Salt-Kala-Namak-7oz/dp/B000JMFCMU/ref=sr_1_8?s=grocery&ie=UTF8&qid=1387793704&sr=1-8&keywords=kala+namak

For all those people who have linseed and flaxseeds growing in their gardens, naturally, they are going to be using these seeds and nuts to get their systems moving. But did they know that linseed and flaxseeds leaves can be made into a delicious dish, like any other green leafy vegetable? This is a great flatulence, preventive, while flax is normally used to prevent constipation

People suffering from enlarged spleens are going to show symptoms like weakness, loss of appetite and a swelling in the splenic region. This can be easily cured by eating horseradish, along with the leaves and black salt on an empty stomach. Try it out now.

Migraine

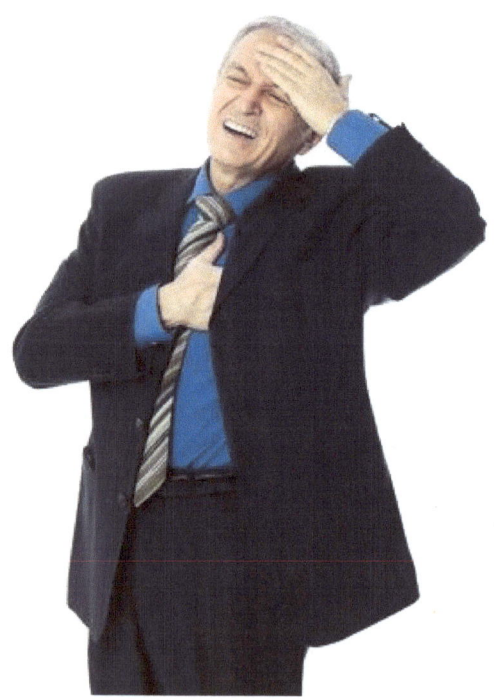

Migraines leave you feeling helpless and miserable. You are also going to feel nauseated.

Now this is one ailment which I would not wish on my worst enemy, having suffered through it, throughout my adult life. Imagine feeling helpless with unbearable pain piercing through half of your head, you unable to see anything, nauseated and no medicine able to give you relief for the next 24 hours. Some people suffer so terribly from migraine that they even consider suicide because they feel that there is a brain tumor growing in their heads. So after a particularly bad attack of migraine which had me wondering whether to apply the family's Webley- Scott revolver or grand uncles's custom made Purdeys (*yep, he had two of them once upon a time…*) to my temple in a *to be or not to be* decision, I finally found out a sure fire cure for migraine.

This is rather amusing and very effective, because it panders to anyone with a sweet tooth.

- Drink half a cup of hot *jalebi* syrup every morning, for a week. You will never suffer from migraine ever again in your life.

For those who are not *au courant* with Indian sweetmeats, jalebi is a sinfully luscious and addictive preparation, which is dumped into thick, concentrated sugar syrup. After five minutes, the jalebis dripping with syrup are taken out and drunk with hot milk. This happens to be the normal breakfast appetizer of all old North Indian rustics in the winter, before they go back home to desi ghee stuffed pancakes. I am not a rustic but I can't resist it with hot milk, now that it is December.

Scientific tip: Could the possible sugar concentration have a physiological effect upon those brain synapses which short-circuit to cause migraine? Tally ho scientists, on the hunt!

Oh, Those Pearlies… (Tooth and mouth care)

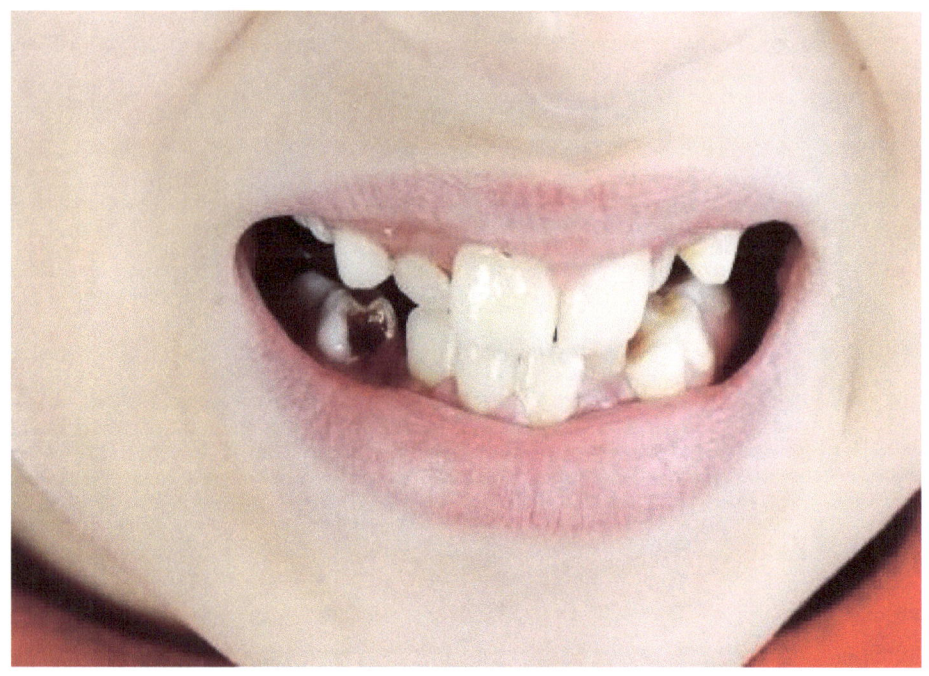

We do not want our teeth to look like this do we?

I spent part of my childhood in Hyderabad, South India, which by the way happens to be the last bastion of rich , cultured and aristocratic feudal traditions brought about by the Persian and Iranian families who entered into the rich Nizam's service. Their beautiful young daughters were married off to the aristocrats of the court. Some of the most beautiful ladies were hidden away in the Nizam's harems and their most exquisite and fragile looking descendants were my classmates at school in the 70s .(St. Ann's High School Marredpally Secundrabad).

In fact, I had 2 of these most exquisite friends, one of them a dead ringer for Walt Disney's Snow White and the other could beat Miss Universe – imagine a light brown haired Tinkerbelle as a baby girl – with one hand tied behind her back, if there was ever a chance of a 7-year-old entering those beauty stakes!

Thanks to their great great-grandmothers, these lovely young ladies would never ever have to worry about wrinkles, bad skin, and bad teeth. Of course some recipes were rather staggering, like using the *Ash of mutton bones in mustard oil*, but I am giving you some of the more innocuous recipes for keeping those pearlies and fangs glinting.

- Collect some oyster shells and burn them. Add salt to the ash and use this powder as a tooth powder.

- For firming up your **loose gums**, massage them regularly with mustard oil, a pinch of soda bicarbonate and rock salt. Let me admit that this recipe was given to me by my grand uncle who has the most beautiful set of teeth in the whole family, even though he is hitting 90. And they *are* really white, like pearls.

- The moment I feel any sort of gum infection coming on, I immediately massage that infected area with a salt/mustard oil mixture. Not only does that disinfect bacteria by getting rid of any bacteria, but it also cures the infection naturally.

- Another relative of mine advocated frying, and then grinding turmeric with salt. This tooth powder was made into a paste with a little bit of mustard oil, and used upon the gums and teeth. As he is still capable of cracking walnuts at the age of 85, this must work, even though I have found it a rather messy procedure!

- To cure **pyorrhea,** make up a powder with these ingredients—

- ❖ 10 g lime paste (*chuna*),
- ❖ 25 g rock salt
- ❖ 25 g alum
- ❖ Three cloves.

Grind these together and put them in a glass bottle. Massaging your gums and teeth with this powder, two times a day is going to remove pyorrhea within 10 days.

These herbal powders are really effective, and are normally made up fresh every morning and sold upon long route buses by salesmen, whose patter could make an Irish showman look to his laurels. The cost is only $0.10, and I bought one for my father, who used it effectively and managed to save his four remaining natural teeth from going the way of all teeth.

And now that I have the herbal recipe, they shall be preserved and protected!

- But what do you do if your **teeth start shaking**? Easy, make up an equal proportions tooth powder of powdered cumin seeds and rock salt. Massage your gums and teeth with this powder two times a day.

- **Ulcers in your mouth** - Now this is one thing up with which I do not put. They can be cured by eating ripe tomatoes and rinsing out of your mouth with tomato juice ever so often. My grandmother also used to feed us a ripe banana in yoghurt to cure the ulcers in our mouths. These normally occur when I have eaten something which does not suit my system, and once I got them by drinking burning hot chicken soup. [Ouch, but I had just come in from the cold, and I did not quite gauge how hot it really was…] * **Mouth ulcers are really painful.**

Try applying pure desi ghee to your ulcers, before you go to sleep so that they can be cured while you are resting. [**Recipe to make desi ghee in appendix.**]

Drooling/Excess salivation

- This is rather a not so amusing part and parcel of growing up for some kids who go around drooling or suffer from an extheth of thalivation. It doesn't seem very funny when you grow up, especially when people make sure they do not get spattered while you are talking away. Mom found out that any normal adult could have this problem if he is dehydrated. So drink lots of water when you hear yourthelf thpitting out your wordth. Apart from that, a tooth powder made of rock salt and Alum in equal proportions will make sure you never emulate your friendly neighborhood pooch.

Toothache powder

Also, cloves have been used through millenniums to get rid of toothache. So the next time your teeth start twinging, especially in the winter, make up a mixture of 1 teaspoon of powdered cloves with 1 ¾ teaspoon of powdered camphor. Brush your teeth with this powder. It is going to keep your teeth, pain-free and trouble-free.

Sensitive teeth

Did you feel a twinge of pain, the moment you bit into something? This means that your nerves in the dental region have grown sensitive. I am going to tell you a remedy, which I use myself, and believe me, the only time I went to a doctor was as a child, and under duress for an annual dental checkup. Add a little ground turmeric to some mustard oil. This is a very strong disinfectant and curative. Rub your gums and teeth with this at night.

You may feel the mustard causing your mouth to salivate. Do not worry, just keep spitting out the saliva until you go to sleep. Early in the morning, wash out your mouth with warm water. Remember not to eat or drink anything after you have applied this tooth curing remedy on your teeth. This is a surefire time-tested and distinctly very beneficial remedy.

Are you suffering from caries? Try rubbing that affected area with onion juice. Of course it smells, but you can try this remedy out in the evenings and at night when you know that your friendly neighborhood gossip and snoop is not going to drop in to borrow a cup of sugar.

The Magic of Face Masks

Face masks have been used as a part of beauty treatment since ancient times.

Ancient Egyptian ladies toned the skin with rose water and milk. Alum was used by Greek and Roman ladies as a toning lotion. The ancient recipes are about as much useful today in making the skin smoother, and firmer. Lines and little wrinkles are removed and a complexion takes on a new luster and clarity.

The surgeon gives you a younger face during face lifts, but because it is a fairly expensive process one can obtain the same benefit of finer textured skin and better skin tone by face masks.

People are under the imagination that teenagers do not need any face masks as the skin is already quite smooth and fiddling with the skin can disturb its texture. But often teenage skin needs cleansing and toning. Anyway we can enjoy making natural products at home. Everyone knows that mayonnaise which is so delicious to eat is a wonderful face mask. Every product which is used in these face masks is good for your skin also.

The frequency with which you use a face mask or the ingredients you have poured into them is the deciding factor for how often you should use them. Your age has nothing to do with it!

In the East, the most often used face mask is the clay one with *multani mitti._* Fuller's Earth.

The *clay face masks* are spread strictly on the skin surface. They absorb the excess oil and the dust particles while they dry. They tighten our skin and they help to stimulate the circulation. Sometimes it causes discomfort to sensitive skins or dry skins. That is why greasy or harshly textured skins benefit more by these masks.

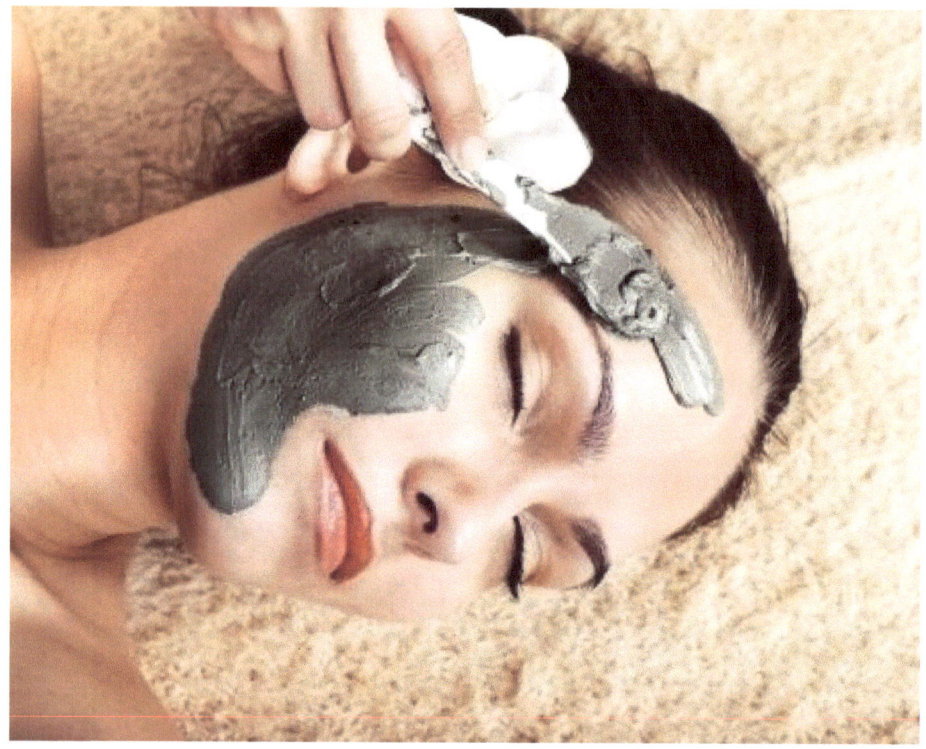

Fuller's Earth is a necessary ingredient in Clay facemasks

The *gel* masks are spread upon a clean skin and allowed to dry. In about 10 to 20 minutes, you can roll it off like a second skin. These masks are peeled off starting from the chin and lifted upwards; you lift out dead cells and even fine facial hairs and sometimes blackheads too with these masks.

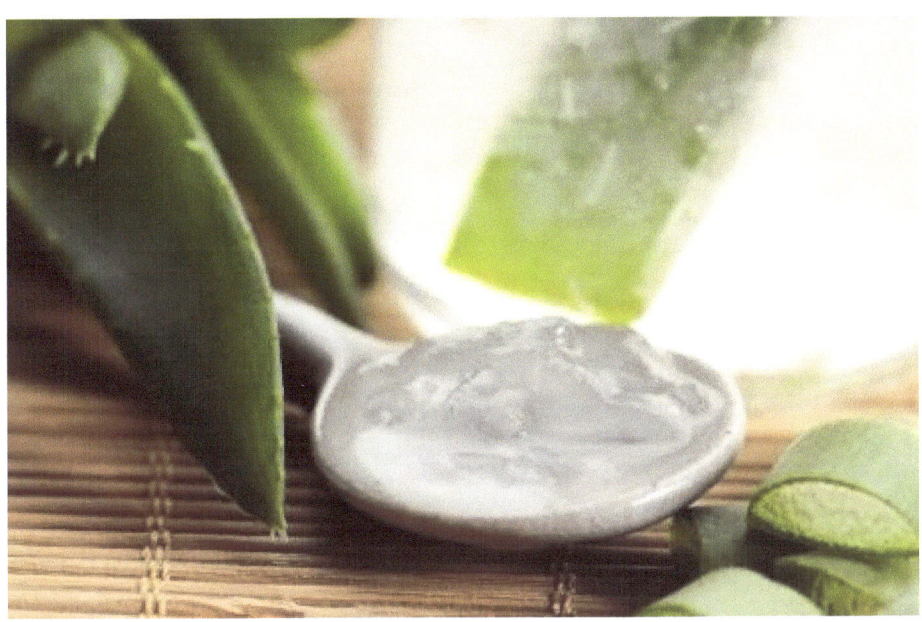

Aloe Vera Gel

These are useful for all sorts of skins from normal to dry and combinations skins but they cannot absorb the body oil like the clay masks can absorb it. In the West, you can find cream type face masks, which have the consistency of thick cream. They feed the skin cells and bring a youthful look back to your skin. They cannot be useful for the young or greasy skins, because they have plenty of oil present in them.

How to Make Your Own Personalized Face Masks

First of all, to experiment upon something start by cleaning your face extremely well. Remote areas of the skin which do not get access to soap and water will have to be cleansed properly. If your skin is dry or normal, put on a moisturizer. I normally use **coconut oil**, because it is natural and it will not prevent the loss of natural body oils with the drying effects of face masks. But if your skin is greasy, go straight to a face mask!

Make sure that you have place to relax, because when you apply the gel or clay type face mask you have to make sure that you keep absolutely quiet for about 10 - 20 minutes. Speaking will stretch out the mask and prevent it from being fully utilized and helpful.

Keep the masks away from the sensitive areas like the mouth or the eyes. Skin here is extremely delicate, and there is the possibility of it being damaged.

Apply a face mask upon the cheeks, forehead nose chin and neck. People normally neglect the neck and it is sometimes very funny to see the face bleached while the neck is still a dusky natural tone! Make sure that the eyebrows are not touched, because if you have a gel mask you don't want to peel off your eyebrows with the mask, do you?

Not that I recommend gel masks or anything chemical. The best ones are of course the natural wonders.

First of all, make sure which skin type you are.

If you have a very oily centre part and dry cheeks, you can use 2 different masks if you want.

Masks for a dry skin

❖ Enough Coconut oil to spread upon your face.
❖ Rose water for after rinse.

Massage the coconut oil in gently. Now take a towel, dip it into hot water, wring it and spread it all over your face. If you lie down the circulation will absorb oil. Repeat this process four or five times and then rinse out your face with warm water. The rose water is to remove all traces of oil. See your skin shine!

Tomato mask

❖ Crush some tomatoes, drink up the juice and spread the pulp all over your face. It tightens up your skin, and closes the pores. The tomato juice is for refining your skin from inside!

Oily skin can be treated with these masks

- ❖ 1 table spoon *Multani mitti.* (Fuller's Earth.)
- ❖ Rose water to make a solution. [Recipe for making rosewater in appendix.]

Spread all over your face if it has blemishes or greasy. In the West the ladies use witch hazel. But in the east , you can always substitute rose water.

What is Fuller's earth?

This article is going to give you more interesting information on Fuller's Earth

http://www.stylecraze.com/articles/benefits-of-multani-mitti-for-face/

Orange mask

- ❖ Half-a-Cup oatmeal.
- ❖ Juice of half orange.
- ❖ Glycerin
- ❖ A little egg white to make a paste.

Beat the egg white and then add the oat meal and juice to it. The glycerin is to moisturize the skin. The egg white gets rid of the wrinkles and the Orange is just to feed the skin. With this mask, open pores and greasy complexions are miraculously rejuvenated .

Normal skins can be treated by these masks

Honey mask

One of Barbara Cartland 's best friend was consider a beauty, because she used to go to sleep with honey spread all over her face. How messy! The best way to use the honey face mask is to dip your fingers into a bowl of fresh warm water and then dip it into the honey which you want to apply to your face. Spread the honey over your face and throat with an upward movement and avoid the eye regions. Let the honey get absorbed into your skin and then wash with warm water. This leaves the skin glowing like pearls.

My favourite is of course, the

cucumber and milk mask

It is wonderful for lighting up the skin, cleaning it toning it and getting rid of all the sun burn.

❖ Take out the juice of 1 cucumber. You can use the pith as extra cleansing material after you have used the face mask. Add the white of an egg, a little bit of milk powder and some rose water for a delicious aroma. The paste is spread all over the face and your neck. This has a wonderful effect upon toning and moisturizing a face, whatever your age is. It is completely natural and has no side effects.

After a face mask it is necessary for toning up the skin, and if you can make a natural skin toner at home why not do so.

❖ Tomato juice is a good skin toner. For normal skin, you can use 1/2 tbs of Alum, 50 grams of rose water and hundred grams of glycerin. Mix them together and put it into the fridge.

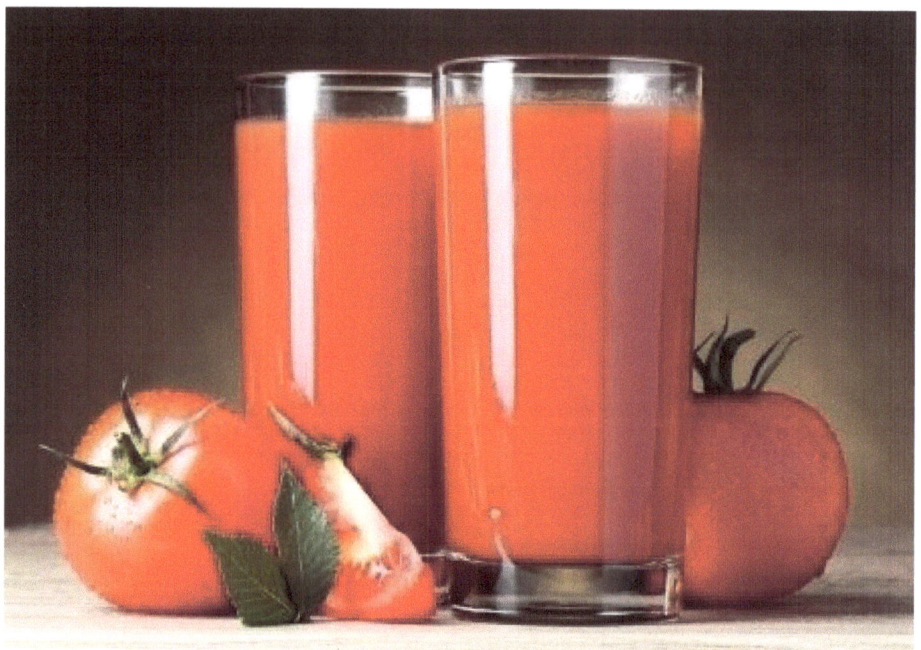

Fresh Tomato juice is delicious to drink too.

❖ For dry skin, boil 2 handfuls of mint leaves in hundred grams of water. This mint extract can be used as an anti-perspirant when you dilute it in water. Mix two drops of it in a cup of distilled water, with half a teaspoon of alum. It is quite refreshing as a Toner applied to a face with cotton wool.

❖ For oily skins, take one teaspoon of alcohol, available at the chemists, with 100 grams of distilled water and half a teaspoon of alum to make a toning solution. Putting it into the fridge helps in preserving it for a longer time, and also a cold toner is wonderfully refreshing when you feel all warmed-up and sweaty!

All these toners are exactly what you get in the market, with fancy labels and high price tags attached, and of course, sometimes they have some chemicals which are detrimental to your skin. The age of a skin toner is for 3 months and that is why preservatives are put into them. But when you make your own, you know what is going into them!

Happy experimenting in beauty masks!

Appendix:

How to make salty lassi to prevent dehydration in summer

1 cup yogurt, 1 cup cold water, salt and pepper to taste. Blend together till it is foamy. Add some ice cubes and give one more whisk in blender. Pour in tall glasses and garnish with mint leaves. This is considered to be the best digestive and is always taken with meals, in many parts of India. In the not, it is called Lassi. In Rajasthan, it may be called chaach and the water content is more. It may be sweet with honey instead of salty. In the rest of India, it may be called Mattha and have spices added to it.

Lassi is delicious with rock salt, pepper, ginger juice, mint leaves, fresh or dry, chopped coriander leaves, salt, cumin seed powder, and even fresh or dry curry leaves. Try experimenting. You may also want to make it sweet. Try this drink in the summer to prevent dehydration. Lassi was considered to be the drink of the gods by the ancients. No wonder they drank it at every opportunity.

Mattha – spicy lassi

Mattha is just lassi with dried cumin seed powder, ginger juice and fresh coriander leaves with salt and pepper. Delicious after a meal, and considered to be an excellent fast working digestive. You may add some water to it. If you think the consistency is too thick, but it is best left alone.

How to make jalebis dripping in sugar syrup

1 cup all-purpose flour

1 tsp besan (chickpea flour)

2/3 cup water.

For the syrup:
2cups sugar
2cups water
Few threads saffron
Cardamom
Oil for frying

- *Combine the flours and yeast in a bowl. Add the water and stir. The consistency should be like pancake batter so adjust water accordingly. Stir till no lumps remain. Let this sit for 20 mins.*

- *For syrup, mix the ingredients in a pot and stir over moderate heat until the sugar dissolves. Increase heat to high and cook undisturbed for 5 minutes. Make sure it does not burn.*

- *Once the 20 mins. are over, spoon the batter into a pastry bag fitted with a plain tube 3/16" in diameter. Squeezing batter directly into hot oil, loop a stream of batter back and forth 4-5 times to form a sort of pretzel . In batches of 5-6 fry the jalebis for 2 minutes or until golden on both sides. As they brown transfer them to the syrup for a minute then place them on a plate. Serve warm or at room temperature.*

In India, sweet vendors spoon the batter into a muslin cloth with a hole through which the mixture can be squeezed. Then they use their wrist action to squeeze the spirals out into one outer circle, one inner circle and the center.

I remember walking down the streets of old Delhi one spring evening to see a very fascinated tourist couple watching jalebis being made in front of their eyes. After admiring the dexterously whirling wrist of the sweetmeat vendor, the girl asked him what it was called. "Jalebi , maddam ji, in English, you are calling it Round Round Stop!"

So enjoy your round round stops, and stop your migraines with its syrup.

How to make Desi Ghee (clarified butter)

Start collecting cream from your daily milk supply. 6 to 8 days, will give you enough of cream to make Desi ghee. Heat the milk cream, and you are going to find it melting into Desi ghee. The leftover sediment is delicious, when spread on Indian breads, Pita breads, or over any spicy dish.

Villagers traditionally make Desi ghee in Asia by adding yogurt to the cream for a week or so. They intend to turn it into buttermilk, fresh butter and Desi ghee by churning. This turning process has three stages. Add water to the yoghurt cream mixture and you get buttermilk and butter. Heat the butter and you are going to get Desi ghee.

Remember to remove the sediment from the top, when you store this Desi ghee in airtight glass bottles. The sediment is delicious on breads with honey. One tablespoonful of this highly concentrated powerful oil spread on every meal surface, including vegetables, pulses and beans – every available visible surface – and eaten every day is considered to be the reason why so many people stay healthy in the villages of Asia. This is, of course, supported with plenty of hard physical work throughout the day.

How to make Rose water (Gulab Jal)

Rosewater is normally available in markets at exorbitant prices, but in India, anybody with access to the red rose – Rosa Damascena -and a little bit of time enjoys making Rosewater at home. This Rosewater is used in cosmetics, as well as in cookery to impart the flavor of the Rose to your meal or to your skin.

Ingredients needed- 1 Cup Rose petals – 12 to 14 flowers.

2 cups water

Lots of ice.

A huge cooking pan – pan number one – with lid in which another pan – pan number two – can be placed comfortably.

Rosewater is just a matter of distillation. Put a wire stand in pan number one, on which you are going to stand the other pan number two. The condensed Rosewater is going to fall into pan number two.

Place the petals at the bottom of the pan number one. Now, cover the petals with water. Place pan number two on the wire stand. Now take the lid and place it upside down on pan number one, thus effectively covering the Rose petals, pan number two and the water. The Rose water is going to condense when you place the blocks and chunks of ice on the inverted lid.

You are going to have a cupful of precious distilled Rosewater, after 25 minutes of slow steaming of the Rose petals.

Precautions – remember to have enough of water to cover the Rose petals. Also, it should not be of such a large quantity, that it displaces the wire stand.

This cooled water is now pure Rosewater. Place it in a sterilized glass bottle. Use it to your heart's content. You may see a little bit of oil swimming over the surface of the water. This is Rose oil, and is even more precious. So if you used lots of petals in a larger pan, you may find even more Rose oil.

This method is for all those people who use a pressure cooker while cooking food. In fact, it is a common way to cook food in Indian kitchens, though I was surprised to see that many of my Australian friends were surprised on being confronted with a pressure cooker for the first time. I told them that pressure cooking the steaks before marinating and barbecuing for just 1 to 2 minutes would make kangaroo meat steaks softer and even juicier. They agree. Anyway, I digress.

You would need water, petals, a pressure cooker and a long thin pipe which it does not melt, when subjected to heat.

Put the water and the petals in the pressure cooker and cover it. Now cover the thin pipe with wet cloth in order to keep it cool. Attach this pipe on the lid of the pressure cooker where you normally attach the weight. Allow the petals to cook slowly, they seem to build up, go through the cooled pipe and collect in a utensil. I tried this way too, but I find the ice on the lid one easier!

Conclusion

I hope you like this second volume of grandma's natural remedies and beauty recipes. This collection is going to keep you healthy and strong, naturally. In fact, these were the remedies which were used by the ancients in order to keep healthy, while they lived through centuries. Methuselah – the grandfather of Noah- lived for 969 years, seven days before the coming of the great flood. Methuselah's father Enoch lived for 365 years. This was due to the excellent diet eaten by the patriarchs. Also, they were not subjected to radiation and pollution. The earth at that time was protected by a canopy of water vapor which gave them their longevity. Also, the people at that time lived a productive and simple life, without bothering much about the stress and tension, which affects mankind in the 21st century.

So it is time for all of us to go back to nature and to her gifts and bounty. May her blessings keep you healthy and well throughout your lives.

Author Bio

Dueep Jyot Singh is a Management and IT Professional who managed to gather Postgraduate qualifications in Management and English and Degrees in Science, French and Education while pursuing different enjoyable career options like being an hospital administrator, IT,SEO and HRD Database Manager/ trainer, movie scriptwriter, theatre artiste and public speaker, lecturer in French, Marketing and Advertising, ex-Editor of Hearts On Fire (now known as Solctice) Books Missouri USA, advice columnist and cartoonist, publisher and Aviation School trainer, ex- moderator on Medico.in, banker, student councilor ,travelogue writer … among other things! One fine morning, she decided that she had enough of killing herself by Degrees and went back to her first love -- writing. It's more enjoyable! She already has 38 published academic and 14 fiction- in- different- genre books under her belt.

When she is not designing websites or making Graphic design illustrations for clients who want Walt Disney, Norman Rockwell , JJ Grandville or Hed Kandy type illustrations, she is busy browsing in old bookshops for antique books,-she has a mouthwatering collection of priceless First editions and rare books…including R.L. Stevenson, O.Henry, Dornford Yates, Maurice Walsh, C.N.Williamson, and the crown of her collection- Dickens "The Old Curiosity Shop," and so on… Just call her "Renaissance Woman" - collecting herbal remedies, making one of a kind creations in Irish Crochet and Aran knitting, acting like Universal Helping Hand/Agony Aunt, or escaping to her dear mountains for a bit of exploring, collecting herbs and plants, trekking, and rappelling.

Check out some of the other JD-Biz Publishing books

Gardening Series on Amazon

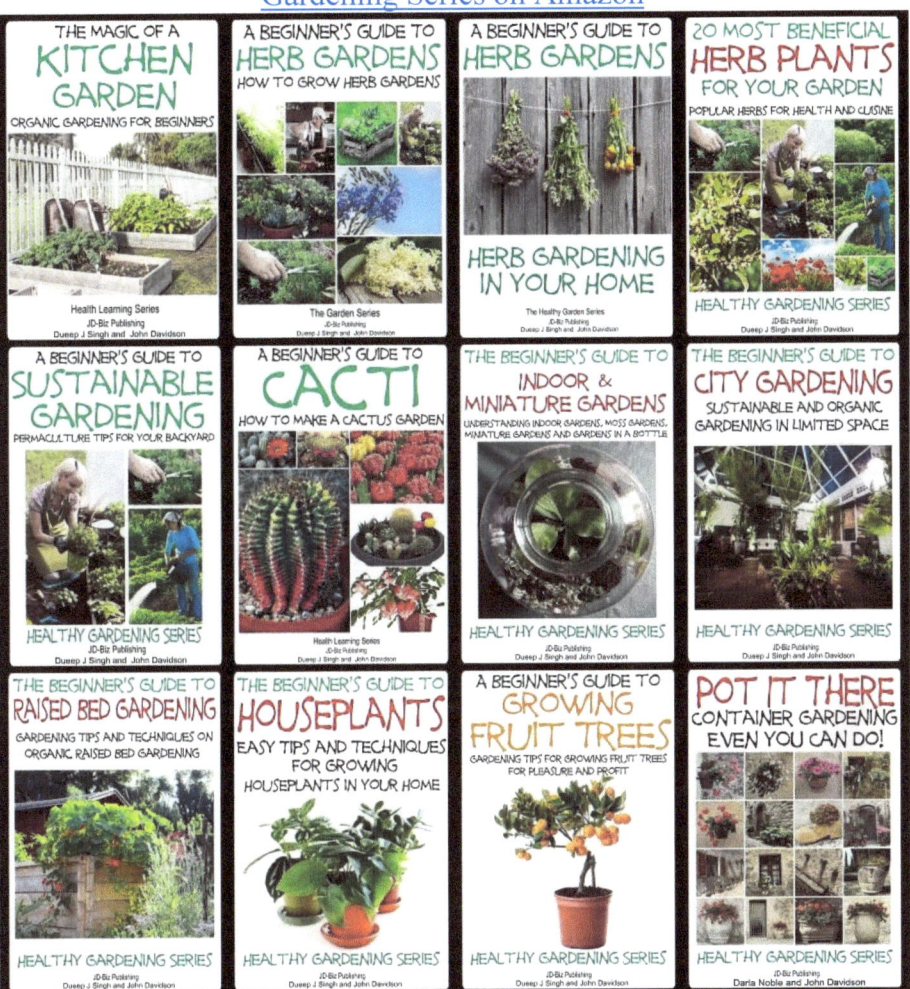

Download Free Books!

http://MendonCottageBooks.com

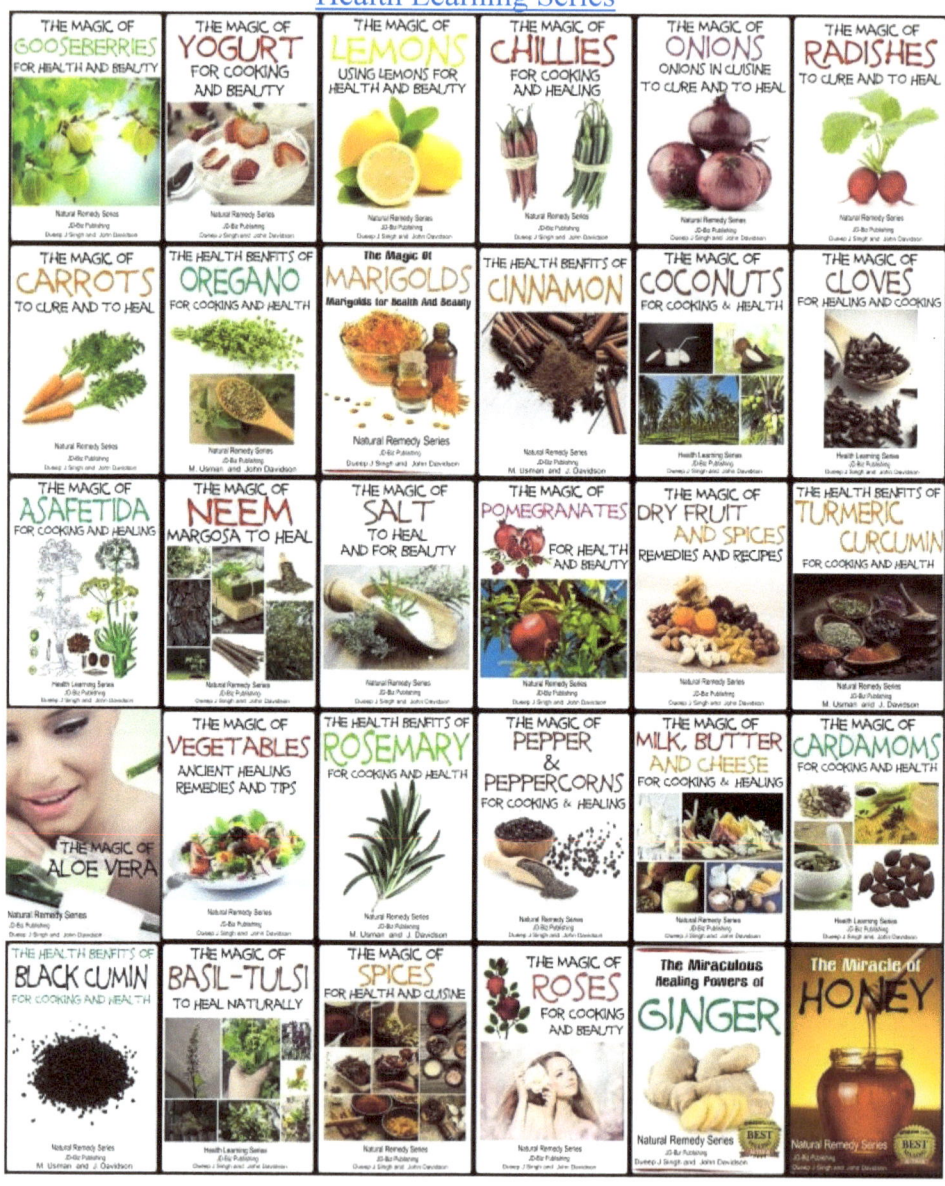

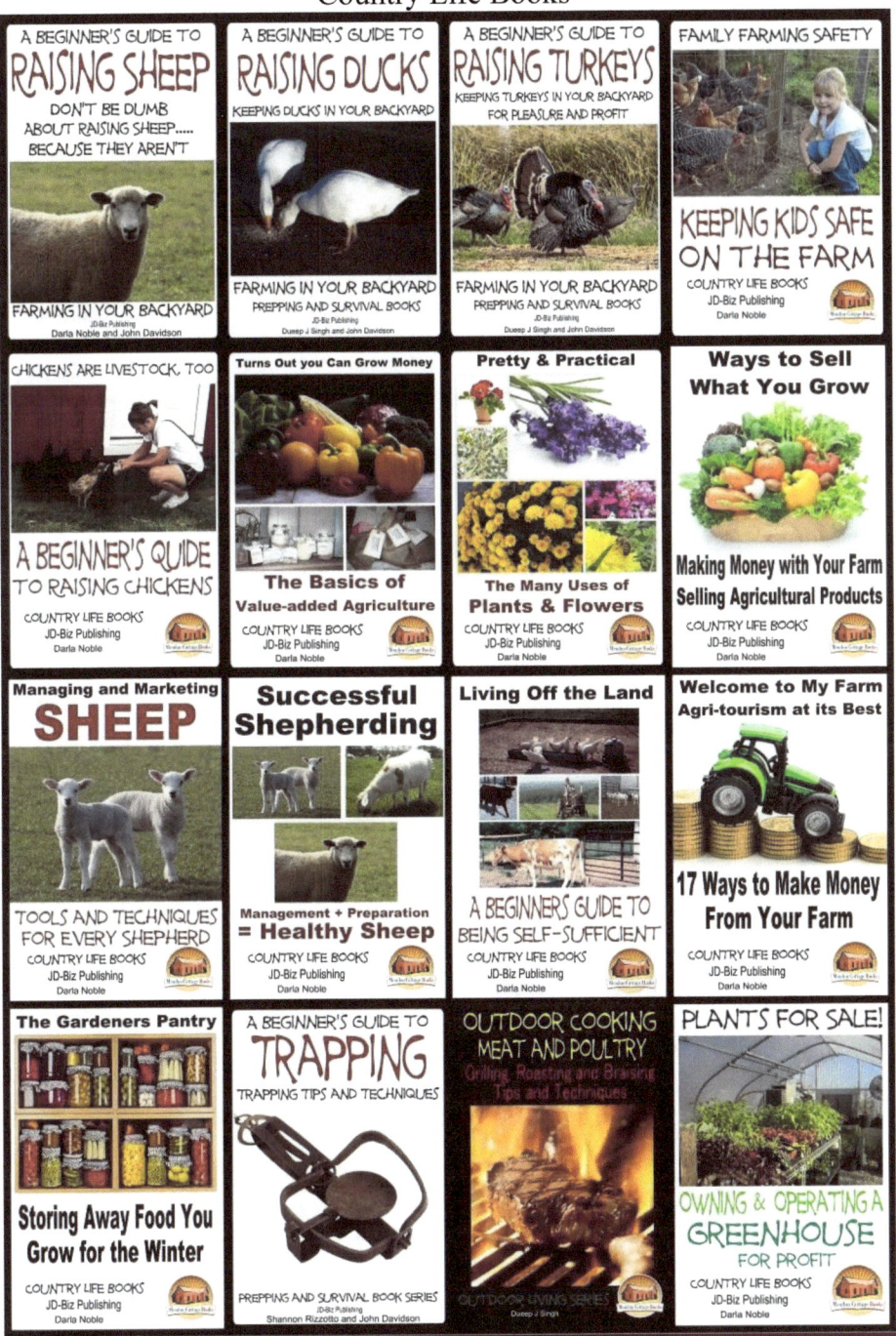

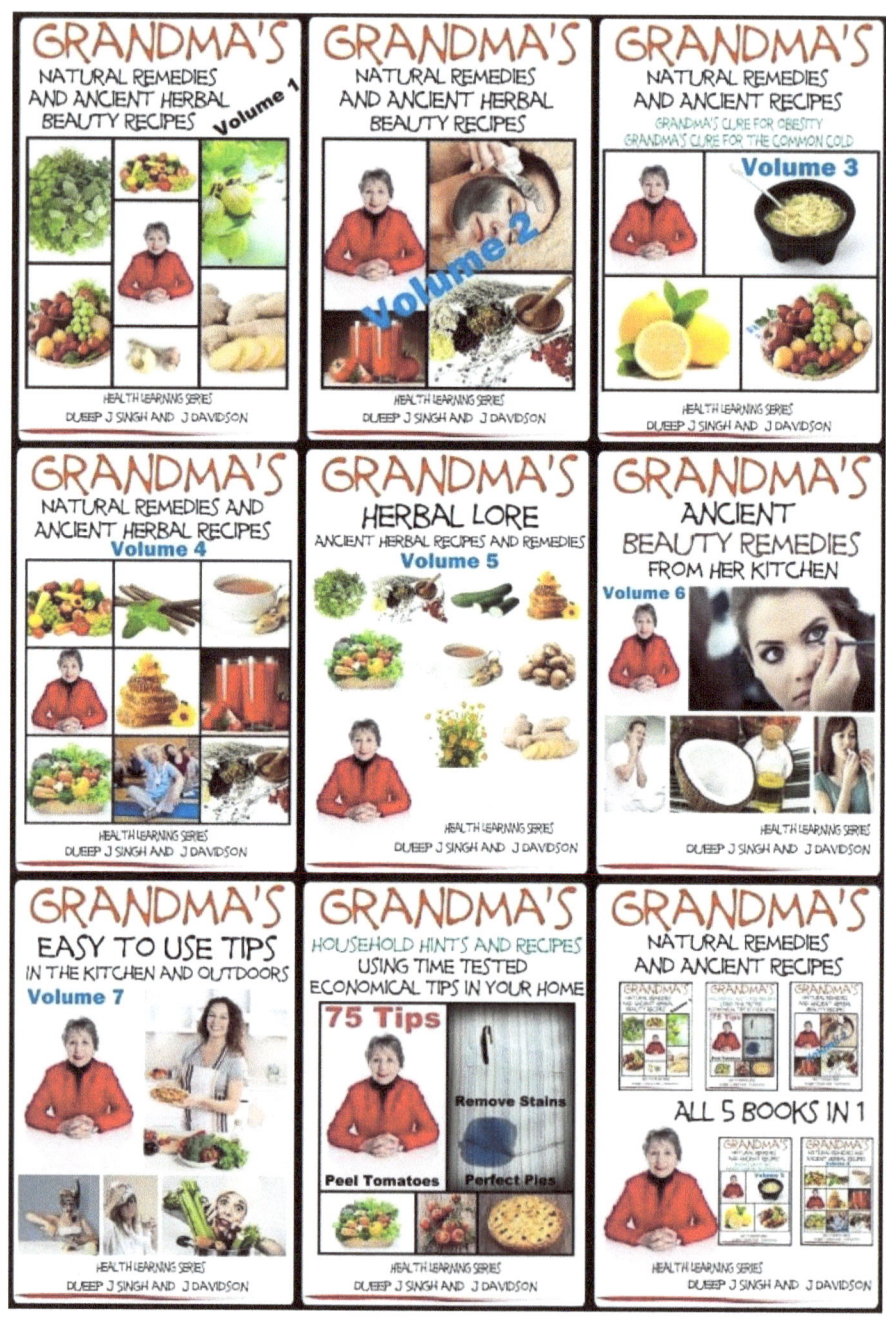

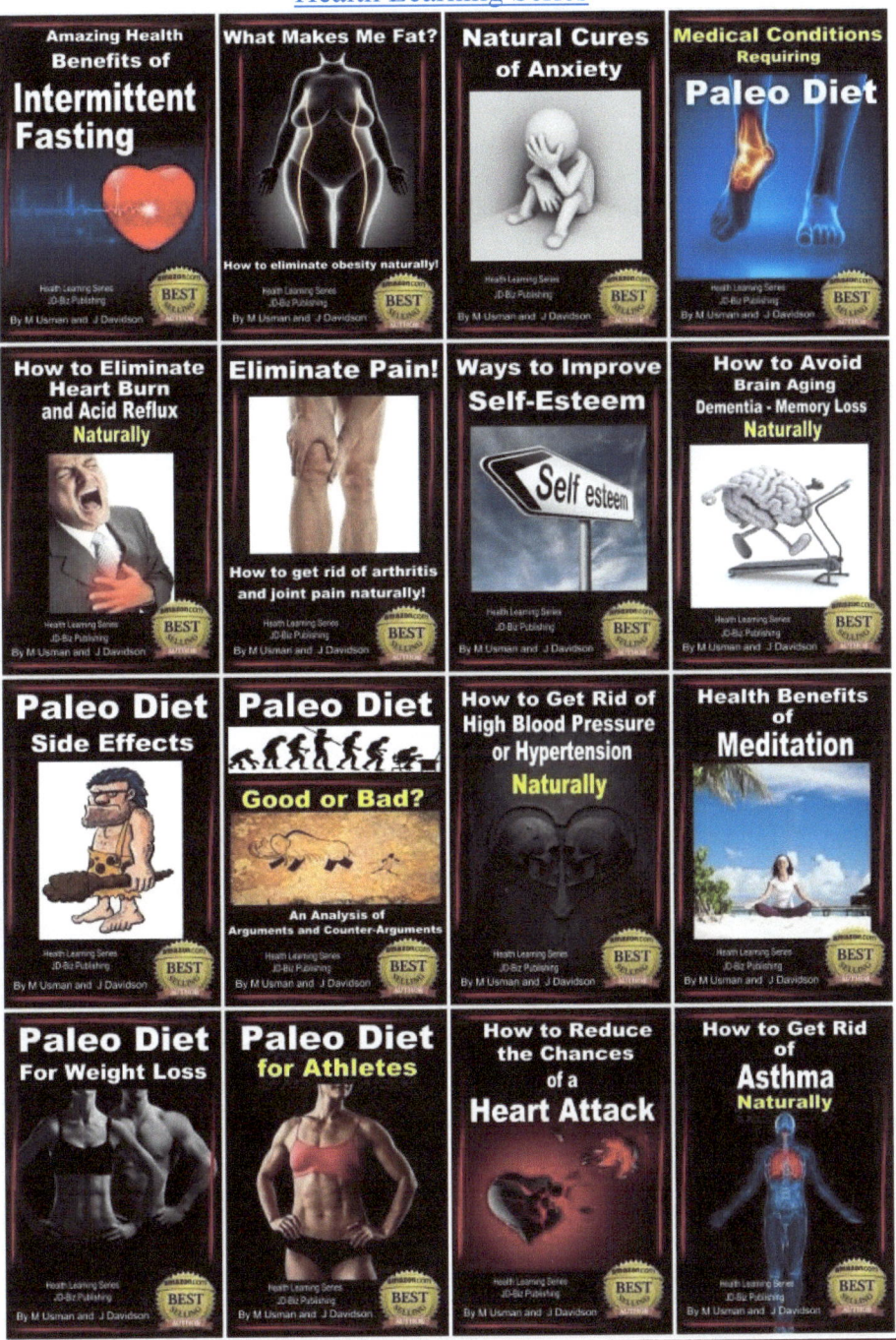

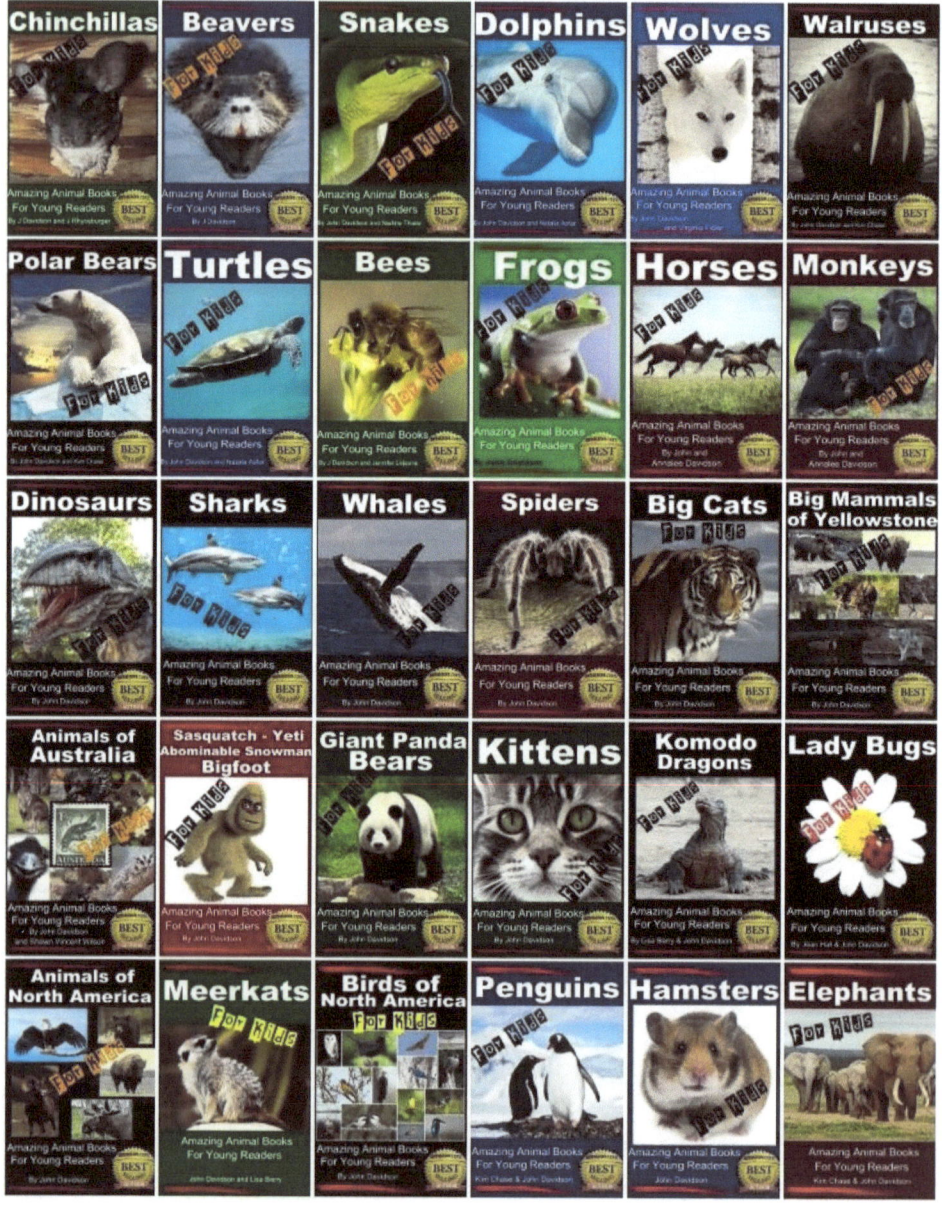

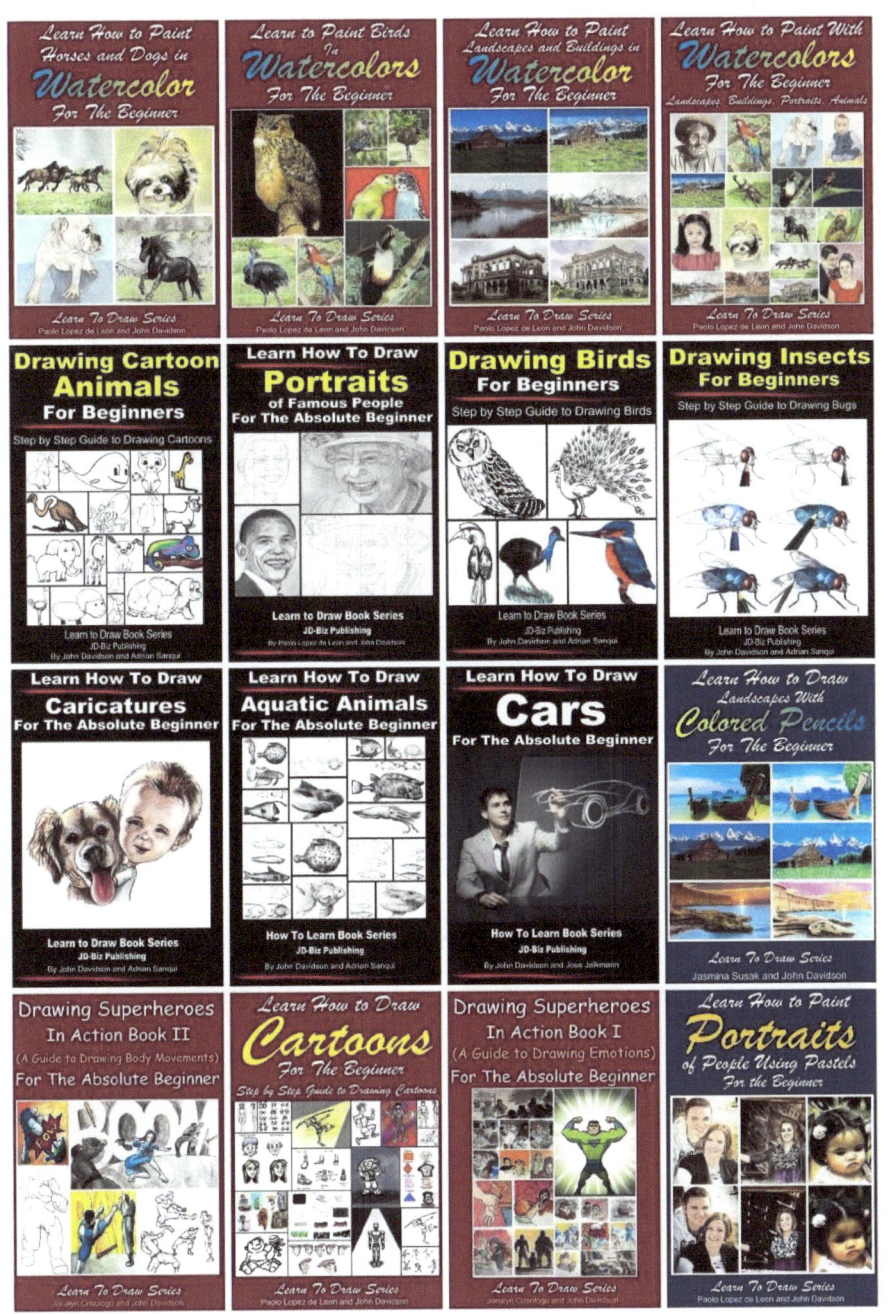

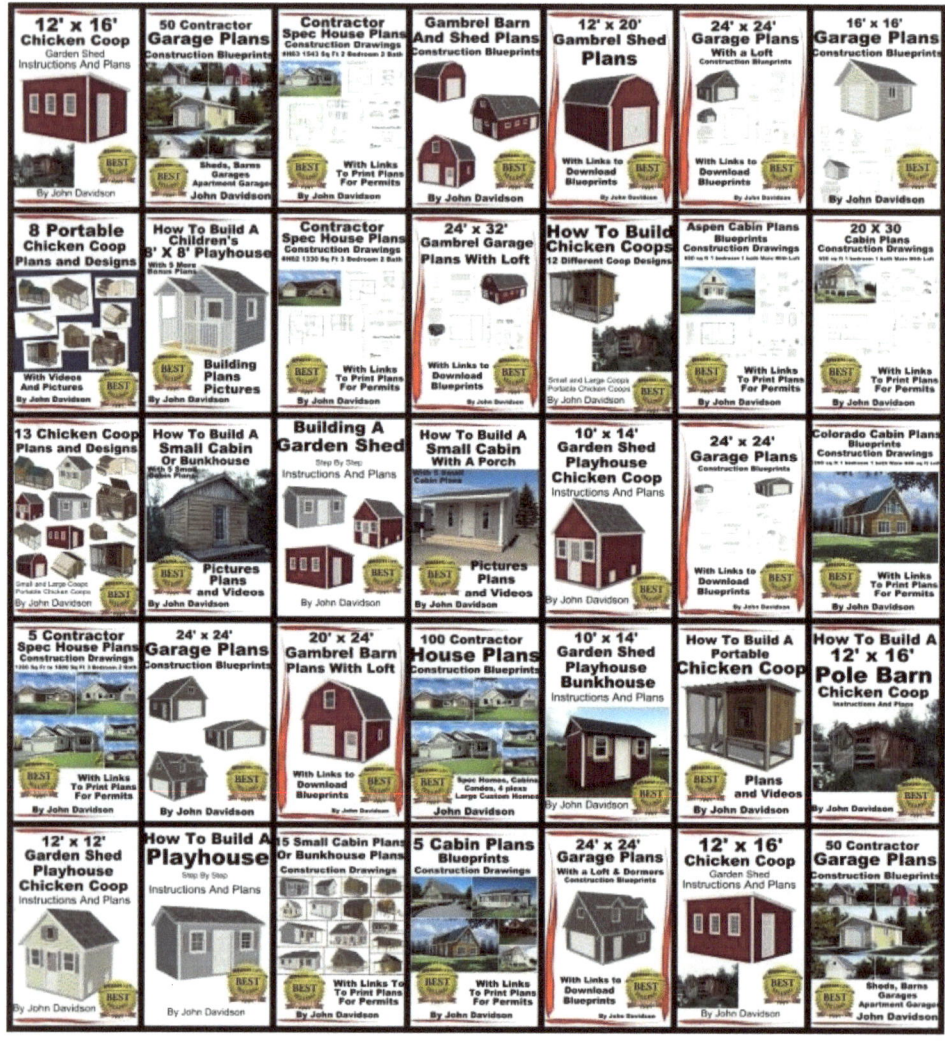

Entrepreneur Book Series

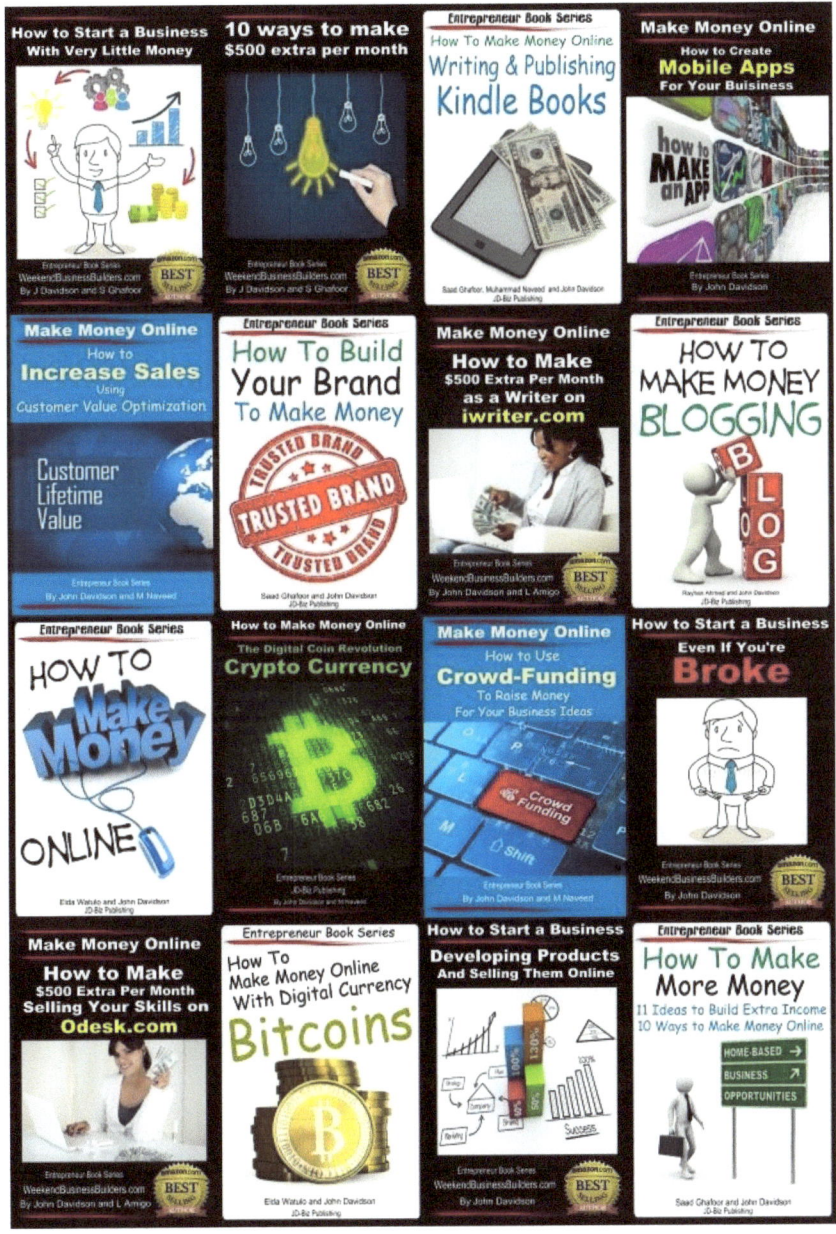

Our books are available at

1. Amazon.com
2. Barnes and Noble
3. Itunes
4. Kobo
5. Smashwords
6. Google Play Books

Download Free Books!

http://MendonCottageBooks.com

Publisher

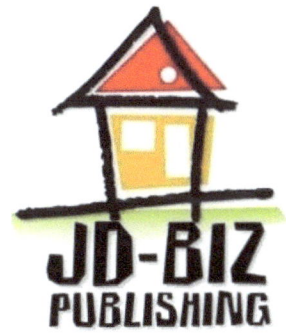

JD-Biz Corp

P O Box 374

Mendon, Utah 84325

http://www.jd-biz.com/

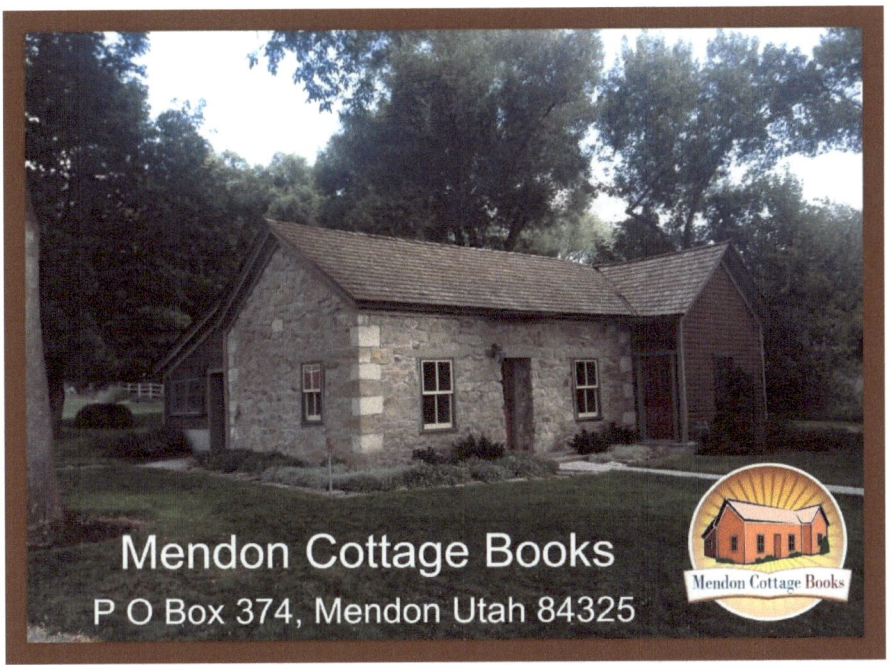